75 Pounds Down Without Exercise

How I Lost Weight, Kept It Off, and You Can Too

Al Haych

Table of Contents

If Man Made It, Don't Eat It

Fitness icon Jack LaLanne, who lived to be 96 years old, and who was working out the day before he died, once said about his diet:

"If man made it, don't eat it!"

If you take anything away from this short book to help you on your weight loss journey, it should be that quote. That's why I put it at the beginning.

Go Down in Size, But Don't Go Up

The second thing I want to mention is about Karl Lagerfeld, the famous clothes designer, who got fat as he got older.

At one point, in his 60s, he decided that he wanted to wear clothes by a particular designer, Hedi Slimane. Slimane's clothes are made for skinny young men.

Lagerfeld spent 13 months losing 94 pounds because he wanted to fit into Slimane's clothes. **Lagerfeld purposefully lost weight without exercise.**

Karl Lagerfeld helped write a book about his journey, The Karl Lagerfeld Diet. If you can find a copy of the book, it's worth buying just for Lagerfeld's motivations. The recipe part of the diet book is a bit ridiculous.

In the book, Lagerfeld provided another good bit of philosophy when he said, **"Go down in size, but don't go up."** I thought that was excellent advice. Never buy a larger size.

Exercise is the Hardest Way to Lose Weight

I've lost weight in the past with exercise.

I'd run 12 miles. I'd swim 5000 meters. I'd get on the indoor cycle and pedal for hours.

Yes, I lost weight.

But it also made me hungry.

It gave me excuses to "cheat" on my diet.

I got injured.

I messed up the muscles around my ankle many times. I lost my big toenail due to stubbing it on the sidewalk while running and had to quit running.

Does that sound like fun?

If only there was a way to lose weight without rigorous exercise.

There is! Re-read the Jack LaLanne chapter, and keep reading!

No Cheat Days

You cannot have "cheat days".

It's like people in AA thinking that they can have a beer or two, but a week later they're getting arrested for Driving Under the Influence.

People think they need constant variety with what they eat.

Where do these ideas come from? Advertising. The Government. Peer pressure.

We're told that you must eat a "balanced diet" of everything in the grocery store.

Or if we eat anything "bad", it should only be done in "moderation".

People say, "Oh, I had steak yesterday. I can't have it today!"

Stop being a princess. There's nothing wrong with having steak a couple days in a row.

Peer Pressure

The office is the worst place for trying to lose weight.

Look around to see how fat everybody has become.

They're holding their Starbucks sugared drinks in the morning.

They eat every couple of hours.

They snack.

Somebody has a birthday, so it's time to break out the cake and ice cream.

The vending machine is always stocked with junk filled with chemical and preservatives.

Even being with friends at a restaurant can be difficult.

"Come on, have some fried chips!"

"Let's share this carrot cake for dessert!"

Most drinks have sugar, chemicals, or alcohol in them.

You want to "fit in" with others, but you can barely fit in the booth.

Family members do the same thing. They'll say: "It's the weekend. It's the holidays. Let loose. Enjoy life."

But it's hard to enjoy life when you're 75 pounds overweight.

The News Is Stress

As you lose weight, you also want to eliminate stressful things.

I quit watching and listening to "The News" many years ago. Even if I pass by a TV, it makes me cringe with stress. I never look at it while on the internet.

Many people I know can't give up watching "The News". They must know what "The News" is, and then regurgitate what they heard or read to everybody around them.

One bit of trickery I see used all the time on "The News" is the use of split screens, which is way of keeping everybody divded.

A person will be on the Left and another will be on the Right and they will be dressed up all fancy.

Women on the TV reading the news might be wearing cocktail dresses at 7am. Who wears a cocktail dress at 7am?

Men reading the news on TV are always wearing suits. You rarely see a man wearing a suit in public these days.

The reason they wear such nice clothes is to give a visual display of authority.

All these people you see on TV are actors. They are having their lines fed to them through a Tele-Prompter. Most are well-paid. If you're well-paid, and don't have any other obvious skills other than looking good in a cocktail dress, you'll be obedient to whatever lines your overlords are having you read to the camera.

Their overlords aren't just the network, but advertisers. Big Food. Big Pharma. Certain companies. The people reading "The News" cannot speak the truth.

The scrolling text at the bottom of the screen was put there to hypnotize you. They want you to keep watching, even when the volume is muted. That's the purpose of scrolling text.

Using these simple methods, the news readers can easily fool the public into believing anything, or get people riled up about some manufactured controversy. We see this all the time with all the excuses to go to war halfway around the world.

It's not just the news. The weather has been corrupted. Every rainstorm is the end of the world. Sports have been ruined with virtue signaling about endless causes and other nonsense we're supposed to accept as real. We're supposed to believe that some elite athletes who earn millions every year is oppressed because of traits they were born with. You must avoid these things.

Fly to another part of the country and watch another local network affiliate and you might as well walk into the suburban McDonald's. Everything looks the same. The homogenization of the media is mostly complete. This is by design.

Stop watching the news. Your stress level will go down.

Giving up this kind of stress is like giving up the bad food that is making you fat, or at least unable to lose weight.

I know it might seem to weird to stop caring about a school shooting that happened 2000 miles away, or reacting to government data that is later found out to be a lie, or whether some criminal you've never heard of is going away for 25 years. You don't really need to know any of this.

It's better to spend time reading the labels on your food and understanding what all of it means.

Food

Most of the food in the stores and restaurants is garbage. Everybody should be more careful with that they eat, but they aren't, and that's why they're fat and sick. They just want convenience.

Many people know that sugar is evil. It was responsible for slavery, but today it brings everybody rotten teeth, diabetes, heart problems, and other maladies.

Seed oils, what is commonly referred to in false advertising as "vegetable oil", aren't from vegetables. The processes for manufacturing seed-based cooking oils are scary and help to create a lot of inflammation in people.

Grains, at least in the United States, aren't any better. They're engineered, sprayed with weed killers and pesticides, and then mashed into something whose sole purpose is to have a long shelf life. Lots of people have gluten allergies because of this.

What do I eat? I could give you a list, but you must learn to make your own list. You must learn to read labels and understand what the label says and what it doesn't say.

The kind of food I eat is usually from the perimeter of most grocery stores, or certain health food stores. I'm not perfect, but I try to learn what the label and marketing says.

My philosophy is that I eat food where, if you left it on a counter for a day without cooking, you shouldn't eat it the next day.

Any food in a bag or package in the store is something you shouldn't be eating. It's full of preservatives, dyes, and other stuff your body hates.

Drugs

I don't drink alcohol. I used to, but I stopped as I got older. I didn't have a drinking problem. Once I realized how alcohol destroys the body, I was done. No more beer or wine or distilled spirits. Alcohol is OK for cooking on camping stoves or as an additive for gasoline, I guess. But not for your body.

We all know smoking cigarettes is bad for our health. Throughout many parts of the United States, marijuana, or even CBD oil, is legal. While I don't think weed should be illegal, I'm alarmed at what that industry has become.

If you're going to smoke marijuana, I think you should be required to grow your own. I don't think there should be stores selling this stuff, and states shouldn't collect tax money on it. I also think products like "CBD oil" are mostly scams.

I've had a lot of people try to tell me that these CBD gummies are great sleep aids. You know what else is a great sleep aid? Being a normal weight. Not being stressed out. Not being insulin resistant. And taking Vitamin B1 and Magnesium Glycinate.

Medical doctors, for the most part, are nothing but state-sanctioned drug dealers. Most doctors are now part of groups affiliated with a local or regional hospital organizations, and they are regularly instructed to push certain medicines on their patients for the sake of profitability and kickbacks. It didn't used to be this way.

If you go in for a routine blood test, chances are the doctor will want to put you on a statin drug. Statins are one of the biggest scam prescription drugs out there, and they have enormous side effects. If you're on a statin drug, do your own research on the history of how statin drugs were developed. Don't talk to your doctor because he or she is likely "on the take".

Ask anybody who works in a medical office about the regular visits by Big Pharma reps bearing sugary cupcakes from the most expensive bakery in town. If your doctor's office refuses the drug company rep's attempt at lobbying and influence, you're likely in the right place.

There are also some recent "miracle weight loss drugs". Semaglutide, often marketed under names like Ozempic or Rybelsus or Wegovy, does work for people who refuse to quit eating garbage. It's also very expensive and comes with side effects like nausea, vomiting, diarrhea, abdominal pain, and constipation. Other than that, I'm sure it's perfectly fine. The FDA approved it. We all know the know the government never makes mistakes.

Or you could simply change what you're eating and how often you're eating it.

My Story

I get sad when I see people who are extremely obese. They could change their life, but they don't know how to do it, or they're given the wrong information.

I am at a normal weight now, but at one time I weighed 75 pounds more than I currently do.

How did I lose weight? I didn't exercise it off. A fat person exercising is the hardest way to lose weight. When somebody is fat and exercising, it is the best time to have an injury.

Counting calories is also dumb. All calories aren't the same, despite what some people say on TV.

To lose weight without exercise, you must be willing to do two things.

1. You must give up most of the foods you used to eat. No more fast food. You must prepare it yourself. No fried food. No sugar. No alcohol. No chemical substitutes. Try to buy organic.

2. You must eat within a limited time period each day. I got to the point where I stopped eating breakfast in the morning. Today, I never eat food before noon. Breakfast is not the most important meal of the day, it's the worst. It's a stupid marketing slogan pushed by a bunch of freaks who run the sugared cereal industry. Stop snacking. Stop going to the vending machine. Just eat around noon and, if you still feel hungry, maybe have a small or limited amount of food around 5pm. And sip lemon water throughout the day. Cut up lemons and put them in a water container with ice.

You'll live. You're not going to starve to death.

Most fat people in the US could survive without eating for a couple of years. That sounds crazy, but it's true. Long term fasting isn't for everybody, but that's how ancient civilization likely survived. While I'm not into long-term fasting, I'd rather just have one meal a day. Not eating for about 23 hours gives my body a long time to rest. My stomach, intestines, liver, and kidneys aren't working overtime to process the endless amount of food going through it.

I have tried to advise and coach friends and family into losing weight, but most don't want to change. Once you reach a certain age, your body starts to fall apart. If you've got an extra 100 or 200 pounds on you, you'll fall apart faster.

While it took me a couple of years to slowly lose those 75 pounds, I can easily say I look 15 years younger. I'm no longer puffy. I feel youthful. I can bound upstairs, two at a time. I have mental clarity all the time. I sleep great. I take no drugs. Nothing! My blood pressure is normal. Pulse is normal. Bloodwork is normal. I haven't had a tooth cavity in years!

Meanwhile, all my friends and relatives are eating statins, taking blood thinners, using a CPAP machine, and are winded just walking up a few stairs. That's no way to go through life!

Some people say, "talk to your doctor", but most doctors just want to give you expensive drugs with side effects. You need to be careful with doctors and avoid the ones who just want to drug you up.

If your doctor's office has fat nurses, or fat people at the reception counter, or a fat doctor, find another doctor's office.

The last person you should talk to about eating and weight loss is a dietician. These quacks always dish out the same stupid advice: follow the Food Pyramid, eat low fat, but it's OK to have all your poisons in moderation. We have a dietician on every corner, but fat people everywhere.

Doctors

Every diet book says to talk to your doctor before changing your diet.

That's like saying talk to your bartender before going to an AA meeting!

There are some doctors I've listened to and read over the years but have never met. They have changed my life for the better, and their videos and books and interviews may help you.

Dr Sten Ekberg on YouTube. He's a former Olympian who is a real teacher and goes deep.

Dr Eric Berg on YouTube. He's a retired chiropractor.
I've never been a fan of chiropractors, but you'll learn more
from him than anybody else about eating and nutrition.

Dr Jason Fung on YouTube and has written numerous
books.

Dr Michael Eades and his wife, Dr Mary Dan Eades have
authored many books over the years about eating low carb
and healthy keto.

Dr Robert Atkins, the founder of the Atkins Diet, is worth
reading. His name got sold and, unfortunately, is on a lot
of bad products in the stores. His haters have ruined his
Wikipedia profile, but Wikipedia in general is a garbage web
site. Read his books and follow his study of "low carb"
back to William Banting in the 19th century.

Dr Uffe Ravnskov, whose book "The Cholesterol Myths"
came out in the 1990s, was an eye opener for me.

Watch the Low Carb Down Under channel on YouTube,
particularly Dr Paul Mason's speeches and interviews.

Education

As I said before, you must learn to interpret the food ingredient labels and understand the marketing terms. You'll get that knowledge by watching the various YouTube doctors, reading books, and ignoring the conventional wisdom that is making everybody fat and sick.

Attempting to change everything overnight may not be a good idea. It took me years to quit Coca-Cola. Today, I can guarantee that I'll never drink another Coke.

Chemical substitutes aren't the answer. The fake sugars haven't made this country slimmer.

Do you know what maltodextrin is? It's in most processed

foods today. Try to avoid it.

What about "natural flavors"? Are they really natural?

Stop thinking that the studies coming out of famous or infamous universities are the last word.

You should know how university researchers get funded, and the decades-long history of deceit pumped out by them.

A lot of studies being published today are the laziest "junk science" imaginable. Do you know the difference between a legit study and a lazy one designed with the outcome and headline in mind?

Be wary of any new, man-made food products endorsed and invested in by billionaires, and being promoted by the "news".

Do Not Use A Scale

The entire time I was losing weight, I didn't use a scale.

Instead, when my clothes got loose, I shopped for new clothes. I always bought the size lower when I fit into it.

I'm a guy who is around 6 feet tall. At my highest weight, my 36" waist jeans were tight. I probably should have been wearing a 38.

After changing what I ate, it wasn't long before I fit into a 34. Then a 33. Then I fit into a pair of 32" waist jeans I saved from a decade back when I was exercising all the time. Those were my "goal" jeans.

One day, I was in a clothing store, and tried on a pair of 31 waist jeans, loose fit. And they fit! I was so happy that I almost cried.

If something smaller fits, buy it!

As Karl Lagerfeld said, "Go down in size, but don't go up."

A few months later, I fit into 30 waist jeans, loose fit. Bought them!

And why they are a little tight, I do own a pair of 29 waist jeans, loose fit. I can close the rivet and they don't look bad on me.

I also was able to fit into "slim" pants and shirts. 31 slim was my first pair of trousers. Now I'm wearing 30 slim. I never thought I'd fit into anything "slim".

My shirts are all Large or Large (slim cut) because I have long arms, down from XL.

I love shopping for clothes now because all the slim cuts are in the clearance rack at cheap prices.

35

People Talk

If you lose weight, people will notice, and they will talk.

Most people did not understand what I was doing. You cannot explain it to anybody, especially those who are struggling with being overweight. Other people may say things that sound hurtful. They may say that you're too skinny when you're simply a normal weight. They will criticize your food choices.

It is best to give general replies to probing questions. I just said I quit drinking Cokes, beer, and eating Cheez-Its, and now I eat more salads. That is true, but that's not the whole truth.

Once you lose weight, you may want to help others. But the truth is that people can only help themselves. They will only change their lifestyle when they're ready. And for a lot of people that change may not happen. Or if they do try, weight loss may not be permanent.

Final Thoughts

I know this is a short book. It's meant to be a spark to help light a fire for others.

You must be willing to change things in your life and to ignore the popular culture, so-called "experts", and conventional wisdom.

You must educate yourself. I cannot do it for you, but I can point you in directions where you can get started.

I don't know everything. Nobody does.

But I lost 75 pounds without exercising, am at normal weight, and I feel great.

I hope you can get back to normal weight, too.

About the Author – Al Haych

This is my first book.

I was inspired by my brother Ed Haych's first book, Dry Drunk Syndrome, a 47-page book released in the summer of 2023 about the attitudes and actions of alcoholics that poison lives.

I'm not an alcoholic, but I ate the wrong kinds of "food" for many years and had trouble losing weight. I've figured out my problems, lost 75 pounds, and feel great.

I may not be the best writer in the world, but I know what worked for me. It wasn't so much a "diet" as much as a change in attitude and actions about eating.

www.ingramcontent.com/pod-product-compliance
Lightning Source LLC
Chambersburg PA
CBHW070748260726
48660CB00007B/3016